Little Kick in the Butt® series

Sometimes we all need a little kick in the butt, whether it's a gentle reminder to step away from the jamocha fudge ice cream or to park at the back of the lot. Men and women across the country face the same dilemma—they want to live active, healthy lifestyles but just don't know where to begin. The Little Kick in the Butt books are the perfect jump-start. These plucky yet practical guides will encourage, challenge, and reward you along your path to good health.

Other books in the Little Kick in the Butt® series:

30 Days to Get Back in Shape

And coming soon:

30 Days to Lower Stress

30 Days to Eating Right

For more information, visit our Web site, www.fulcrumbooks.com.

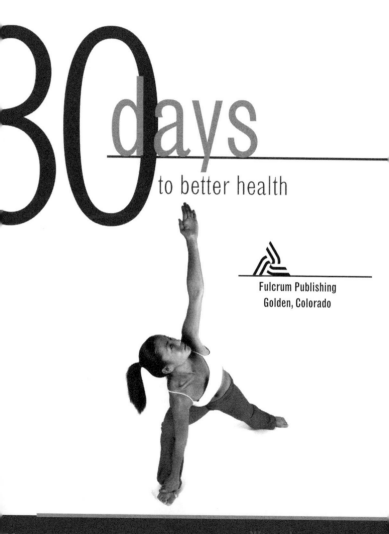

Little Kick in the Butt

30days
to better health

Fulcrum Publishing
Golden, Colorado

Michelle Theall founder of Women's Adventure

Library of Congress Cataloging-in-Publication Data

Theall, Michelle.
  30 days to better health / Michelle Theall.
     p. cm. -- (The little kick in the butt)
  Includes bibliographical references.
  ISBN-13: 978-1-55591-570-4 (pbk.)
  ISBN-10: 1-55591-570-1
  1. Health--Popular works. 2. Health--Miscellanea. I. Title. II. Title: Thirty
days to better health. III. Series: Theall, Michelle. Little kick in the butt
  RA776.T424 2005
  613--dc22

                                  2006014939

Printed in Canada by Friesens Corporation
0 9 8 7 6 5 4 3 2 1

Editorial: Haley Groce, Faith Marcovecchio
Cover and interior design: Jack Lenzo
Cover image: istockphoto, Phil Date
Author photo: Blake Little

Fulcrum Publishing
16100 Table Mountain Parkway, Suite 300
Golden, Colorado 80403
(800) 992-2908 • (303) 277-1623
www.fulcrumbooks.com

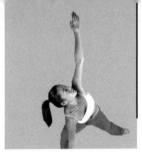

Contents

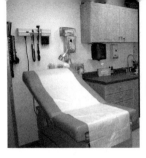

Introduction
How to Use This Book

Picture yourself in the doctor's office, sequestered in an exam room. You sit, hands folded, then pick up a magazine and thumb through, not really reading anything. You notice the walls of the room. They're robin's-egg blue, meant to reassure. Yes, you feel fine. It's just a normal checkup, after all. Nothing to worry about. The doctor returns. She sits on the stool and spins around to face you. Her eyes are serious. "You're dying," she says.

"Dying?" Perhaps your hearing is going too. "That's not possible. How? Why?" You shake your head.

"I've checked with experts in every field. There's nothing that can be done."

"How long do I have?" You're thinking about trips you need to take. People you want to tell that you love them. Your kids, spouse, parents, and friends. Skydiving.

"Well, while some things are out of our control, there are things you can do to prolong what life you have left. Eat right, exercise, lower your stress, take your vitamins, lose a little weight, and make sure you're well rested. Monitor your health."

"Okay," you resolve. "Yes. I'll do it all. Anything I can. Starting today. So, how much time will that buy me?"

"Well, according to the test results, we found that you are a normal human being. So, I'd say anywhere from one hour to 60 years."

We're all dying. We're mortal beings with no guaranteed expiration date. Yes, you may get hit by a bus tomorrow. But maybe not. There are so many things within your direct control that can lengthen your life and make you feel better while you're here. To live life to its fullest, we need to be healthy and nourished in our bodies and souls. Most of us would like to be healthy and happy, but we don't know where to start, what to do, or how to stick to a long-term program. The Little Kick in the Butt series is designed to help you achieve your goals and live a happier, healthier, and more fulfilled life—one day at a time.

Using daily motivations, lessons, and challenges that really work, you'll find yourself in better health after just 30 days. No kidding. Thirty days. "But I've spent at least 30 years spiraling into poor health," you say, "so how can one little book get me healthy inside and out in just a single month?" Well, each day reveals a new way of thinking (little kicks) about food, exercise, and your body. Allow each chapter to become a lifetime habit, and the book will transform you completely. There's no magic pill or exercise that can prolong your life, but changing your lifestyle day by day to incorporate healthy activities will help you enjoy the journey for as long as possible. Embrace the tasks presented in this book, and you'll be on your way to a new and better you.

A few suggestions before we get started:

1. See your doctor. If you haven't had a regular physical in the last 12 months, we recommend that you do so. Consider this checkup the starting point from which you will gauge your progress.

2. Consider asking a buddy or family member to work through this book with you. A support system is always helpful. Plus, you'll have someone with whom to share your insights and celebrate your renewed health.

3. Start out each morning by reading one chapter. I know you're busy, so each chapter will take less than five minutes of your time.

4. Commit yourself to the challenge of the day. As the band U2 sings, "There is no failure here, sweetheart/ Just when you quit." I promise you'll be successful if you commit to doing our daily task. I've done my best to make each day innovative, unique, and fun.

5. Be flexible. Alter the challenge if it doesn't work with your specific situation. For example, if you work from home and the daily challenge is to park in the furthest parking space to get in a few extra steps while walking to your office, you'll have to be a little creative.

6. Avoid burnout. You may be tempted to repeat a daily task and incorporate it into the entire week or month when the challenge doesn't specifically ask for this (sometimes it will). It's understandable to want instant results and get overzealous when something works, but this book was designed to prevent you from burning out by using a more gradual approach. Remember the Atkins diet? People loved their steak and eggs at first, but they soon missed those beautiful and delightful carbs. All or nothing is pretty tough to achieve. Your health is a marathon, not a sprint, so we'll take things day-by-day and step-by-step.

Finally, remember that the status of your health is determined by mind, body, and spirit. We'll be tackling all three in this book.

That's it. Get excited because, starting tomorrow, you're on the road to better health. See you in the morning.

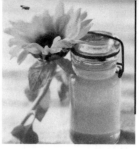

Day 1
No Pain, No Gain

When I was four years old, I decided to pet a bumblebee. My sister shrieked and ran from her swing to stop me. All I could think was that I'd need to hurry and grab the fuzzy ball if I was to know what it feels like to hold it, all soft and furry in my hands. I've deposited that moment, though at the time brief and painful, into the positive side of my memory bank. I like to think that I'm one of the few people in this world who knows what it feels like to pet a bumblebee, and I'm guessing that's something worthwhile. I've come to believe that the bee and my early connection with it are symbolic of the way we all face adversity. We step into life with playful curiosity, sink into the soil on our elbows for a better look, and then—wham! How we rise from the sting determines our character.

Throughout my life, I've attempted to make peace with a lot of "bumblebees." I've been abused, assaulted, and carjacked at gunpoint. I've teetered on the brink of bankruptcy. I've been trampled by a horse and knocked to my knees by lightning. I consider myself lucky and figure, at the very least, I have some great stories to tell.

I was confronted with the biggest sting of my life when I was diagnosed with multiple sclerosis (MS). Traditional medicine didn't work for me, so I decided to approach my battle with the disease as an athlete preparing for a race. Many of the thoughts and techniques in this book were part of my "tough love" program. I share these things because most of us don't think about being proactive until the unthinkable happens—until we get stung. Building a healthy body isn't just a lesson for those with disease, illness, or injury, it's for everyone digging around in the garden of this life. Your health is a giant bumblebee, and it's well worth the risk of becoming friends with it.

Your decision to read this page, simply to start, means that you are ready to take the first of many steps toward a lifetime of better health. You're reaching out your hand and believing the reward will exceed the sacrifice. Petting the bumblebee takes courage. It's been 35 years since I held the buzzing furball in my hands, yet I still write about it. I'm reminded that the best things in life are usually worth the momentary sting.

Challenge #1

As you take your first steps toward a healthy life, you'll be walking a whole lot more. Today, select the farthest parking spot from the grocery store, your office, the post office, the bank, and everywhere else you go.

Why It Works

Americans, fit and otherwise, are quite obsessed with our "good parking Karma." We feel we're being rewarded or that we've outsmarted the universe when we find that elusive and coveted space right in the front row. The truth is, we need those extra steps. Embrace them. On a busy day, they may be the only exercise you get. Plus, you'll lower your stress levels. Just think, no more frantic searches or urges to steal a spot from the minivan driven by a mother of two who turns out to be your neighbor. Need three more reasons? No more door dings. Less traffic. Plenty of room to load and unload your car.

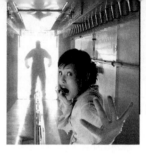

Day 2
Keep the Boogeyman at Bay

It's the classic horror-movie sequence. A girl, the one with the toe-curling scream and big boobs, remains the sole survivor at the abandoned cabin in the woods. Her friends have all disappeared, one by one. She knows they're all dead. There's a diabolical maniac, an escaped murderer from the local prison, running crazy through the forest. He is seven feet tall, carries an axe, and covers his disfigured face with a hockey mask. She trembles as the phone rings. She answers it. The voice says, "I can see you. I'm a killer. I know what you did last summer." Which roughly translates in horror-movie speak to "I'm in the room. Instead of running, grabbing a weapon, or calling the police, why don't you open every scary door and let me get you." There's a noise. Thumping from a killer's bloodthirsty heartbeat. It seems to be coming from the old camp kitchen (where all the big knives are). The girl approaches the door. The camera pauses on the doorknob as her shaking hand reaches toward it and the lights flicker and dim in time with her breath. Should she open the door? Of course not. Will she? You bet.

It's in our nature to investigate and explore those things in front of us. Temptation and curiosity get the better of us almost every day. It's human nature. Temptation is a killer, and we live with a big one. It doesn't wield a knife, but it does tend to hide in the kitchen. Not to worry, though. Exorcism is easier than you think.

Challenge #2

Quick. Name two things you eat every day (perhaps several times a day) that you know aren't good for you. They might be high in calories, filled with refined sugars, loaded with saturated fats, or fried in grease. An item might be a category, such as chocolate, alcohol, fast food, or bread. Or it could be a singular demon, like the cream cheese–covered bagel you have every morning for breakfast or your nightly affair with Ben & Jerry's ice cream. Take a deep breath. Walk to the pantry and refrigerator. Remove the offending items and put them in a bag. Give the bag to the homeless man or woman who sits on the corner you pass every day. Not that the homeless don't deserve good nutrition, but there's just no sense in wasting food.

Why It Works

Temptation is all around. Your office has a vending machine, and the company celebrates every employee's birthday with cake and ice cream. Your daughter is a Girl Scout who swears that if you don't buy 15 more boxes of Thin Mints, she won't win an iPod. Clearly, some situations are unavoidable. But your home can be a sanctuary. Start there. If you have the choice between a shiny apple or a Hostess Cupcake, you'll choose the cupcake every time. Try to remember the psycho killer in our horror-movie scene above. It's bad enough if you bump into him in a dark alley, but you don't have to invite him to come live with you. Cleanse your home from temptation, and you'll be eating better in at least one location. Try to avoid your two vices until later this month (Hint: There's a cheat day or two coming up).

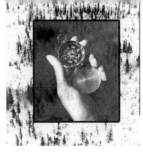

Day 3
Lost in the Wilds of the Grocery Aisle

It's the middle of winter. You decide to snowshoe up to a glacier-fed, frozen lake to have lunch. At least six inches of fresh powder arch the limbs of the aspens into gentle bows. Their arms form a silent canopy, and you cross beneath them. The only tracks you see are those of rabbit and elk. No noise, just peace.

About an hour into your hike, snow begins to fall. It floats to the ground and blends into a white blanket. You sigh into its beauty.

Thirty minutes later the snow blows sideways. You look behind you. The path has disappeared. In front of you, the mountains evaporate into mist and clouds with no distinction between them. In the whiteout, you turn around to return the way you came. Though you can't see the trail anymore, you know you are headed in the right direction.

One hour later you are startled and thankful to see footprints. You call out. No one answers. Yelling again, you look down and notice that your snowshoe fits perfectly into the track you've found. You have been walking in a circle for over an hour.

When blindfolded, adults will walk in a circle and believe they are traveling in a straight line. Our senses can fail us, but our knowledge can save us. For example, using a compass during a blizzard can quite simply save your life. The same can be said about food. Our sense of taste may tell us that something we are eating is "good," but the label may point out just how lost we've become.

Challenge #3

Head to the grocery store today (after you've had a small snack or meal). Remember the items you threw out or gave away yesterday, and avert your eyes from them. They will no longer fill your cart. Everything else is fair game, as long as you read the label first and make decisions accordingly. The goal for today is to get educated about what you are putting into your body. If an ingredient stumps you, look it up online. In general, if it has more than two syllables or can't be pronounced on the first try, it's not something you should eat.

Why It Works

Information is your compass. When you are lost, you ask, "Where am I?" When you eat, you should ask, "What is this?" It's tough to continue eating something when you've found out that it comes from the small intestine of a rat or that the same chemical found in your soda is also a good tar and glue remover. Saccharin caused very skinny and svelte cancer-ridden mice. What's the cost of fitting into a size-two dress? It might be your life. Read up before you eat up.

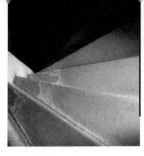

Day 4
One Step at a Time

Cindy Chupak, the award-winning writer and producer of legendary sitcom hits including *Sex and the City* and *Everybody Loves Raymond*, found that biking helped her solve script problems. Chupak's high-stress job had her living on two coasts and working like a madwoman to create shows that touched viewers and made them laugh. When the pressure became too much, she'd hit the road on her bike. "I've taken several bike trips that I've loved," Chupak said, "through the wine country in Italy, across the South Island of New Zealand, and over mountain passes in the Canadian Rockies. There's nothing like the feeling of reaching the crest of a hill or peak and sailing down the other side."

Just as she broke down a ride by each hill and mile, she worked through tough work assignments by analyzing each component. "I've solved so many script problems on the bike path, just thinking about what I want to see, playing the episode in my head," Cindy said. "I've learned on bike trips that you can get over any hill if you break it down, take it a little at a time, and don't dwell on how much you have to do. This is a lesson I carry with me when I grow overwhelmed with work; because even though I love my job, when I have a book to write or 20 episodes ahead of me to script, it's the same as a mountain pass. I get through it the same way—a little at a time."

As a whole, problems may seem daunting and insurmountable, just like a ride across Tuscany. Taken piece by piece, the miles fade in the rearview window.

Challenge #4

Where are you in your steps toward fitness? Do you walk three times per week or swim five laps per day? Perhaps you're just getting started now? Wherever you are, take a moment to evaluate yourself. What is the next step for you? Fitness and health begin with a single step and progress into life-changing habits. Starting now you will add one increment into your current fitness program. For example, if you walk three times per week, make it four. If you swim five laps per day, make six your new routine. If you have no fitness program in place, try a brisk one-mile walk today, and commit to doing it three times per week.

Why It Works

If you are trying to lose 100 pounds, it can be overwhelming to think about how far you have to go to achieve that goal. It would be easy to get into self-defeating mantras and tell yourself that it's just not possible, that you'll never be able to lose all of that weight. But what if you only looked at losing a single pound this week? That seems doable. It's a bet you'd be willing to take.

Breaking a goal down into progressive increments is more than just a psychological boost, it's a physical one as well. All of your muscles, including your heart, get accustomed to a certain level and type of activity. Muscles only grow stronger from being broken down and then, during rest, being rebuilt by the body. At a certain point, your body no longer breaks down muscle, because the exercise is no longer new to it or strong enough in intensity. Push yourself to the next level, and you'll achieve greater results.

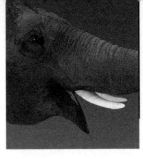

Day 5
Write Your Way to Better Health

Have you ever considered just how odd an elephant looks? It's as if the magnificent giant got assembled at a leftover-parts factory. His ears resemble huge, gray, half-opened parachutes; he's got a tail shaped like a three-year-old's scribble and an itsy-bitsy mouth the texture of candy wax lips from Halloween. As strange looking as the elephant is, we can memorize how he looks, walk away, and later draw him from memory to accurately illustrate what an elephant is to someone else who hasn't seen one. But how would a blind man describe an elephant?

If his hands grasp the trunk, he's apt to tell you that an elephant is a snake. The tusk: a smooth, marble spire. The foot: a tree trunk. His opinion, while correct, won't accurately describe the entire elephant. The man gets part of the picture, but without running his hands over every inch of the beast—a monumental task—or regaining his sight, he'll remain mostly in the dark about this complex creature. He'll need you to tell him about the elephant.

Wellness is an elephant, and we are blind men. Just like the elephant, your health is made up of numerous intricate, tangled, beautiful parts. Often it's impossible to grasp much beyond a single component of your personal health. For example, you may know that you get the hives a couple times per year, but never put that together with an allergic reaction to guava juice. Perhaps you cry every winter, but you don't realize your sadness results from a lack of sunlight.

If we could see a doctor or psychologist every single day, we'd have a complete and detailed record of our mental and physical health. We'd have impartial people to put the pieces of our health together into a picture we can understand. Since that's not practical or financially feasible for most of us, we need to become an objective viewer of our own health. We need to back away from the elephant to see beyond one part of its whole. By keeping a health journal, we can distance ourselves enough to become analysts and begin to see our well-being in an entirely new and illuminating light. Through the pages of your journal, you can begin to understand something complex and magnificent: YOU.

Challenge #5

Start a health journal today. This notebook will be a daily record of your mental, physical, and spiritual well-being. Make your first entry this evening. Be as creative as you want to. This is your diary and no one else will ever see it. For starters, tell what you ate today, what type of exercise you did, and how you felt overall.

Why It Works

Objectivity is key. By keeping a health journal, you can look back and see important patterns you might otherwise miss. For example, your PMS was better in the months when you remembered to take your vitamins. Or you slept better and woke better rested on the days when you sat in the whirlpool for ten minutes. At the end of each entry, you may even be surprised what you've been hiding from yourself all these years.

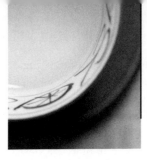

Day 6
Soup's On ... and On ... and On ...

We've all heard the saying "Your eyes are bigger than your stomach." Roughly translated, this means that we order more than we can eat. Wrong. If the bowl remains full, we'll just keep right on eating. As reported in the 2005 Obesity Research report, researchers conducted a study telling subjects they were going to be part of a taste test. They gave a control group a normal portion of soup, while the test group in a separate room received a bottomless bowl (one that continued filling from underneath the table as soup was consumed). The result: The test group consumed 73 percent more soup than the control group.

We've been conditioned to eat everything on our plates. From childhood we were told to be ashamed for wasting food. To be exact, "There are hungry children in Ethiopia, or China, or Russia." We've become a nation of plate-clearers, and our waistlines show it. The funny thing is that in this particular study, the control group reported being just as sated as the test group and believed they had consumed the same number of calories. Eating more didn't result in any greater satisfaction. In fact, personal experience proves the exact opposite to be true. Continuing to eat until we feel full leaves most of us past the point of comfort. We pay the price with bloating, stomach cramps, gas, and indigestion. Nothing can tarnish the culinary delight of fine dining more quickly.

Challenge #6

Today's focus is on food portions. All day, take every meal or snack and cut it in half before you start eating. Box the other half and save it for lunch, dinner, or for other family members.

Why It Works

Half the calories. According to researchers, you may not even miss them.

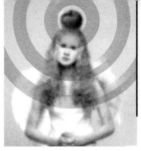

Day 7
Eve Was Set Up, Baby

Never and *always*. Wow. Those are two loaded words. Responsibility. Guilt. Forbidden fruit. Never and always set up unrealistic expectations. I will never eat chocolate again. I will always exercise every day. This is unrealistic, not to mention boring. Discipline is an important character attribute, but taken too far, discipline turns into obsession. Why did Eve eat the apple in the Garden of Eden? I'm guessing at some point she became obsessed with it. Perhaps she even ate the entire tree of apples after being forbidden to eat them at all. Then she had to join Weight Watchers, and Adam threatened to leave her because she started to get round and flabby. All that from always and never—not to mention original sin. Whew. Who knew?

Theological kidding aside, researchers at Pennsylvania State University actually tested the theory of forbidden fruit on groups of three- to five-year-olds. The children were asked to rate various food items including cheese crackers, peanut butter crackers, chocolate chip granola bars, apple bars, peach bars, and strawberry bars as "yummy," "yucky," or "just okay." As the researchers made certain items less available to the children, they found the children craved those items all the more. In fact, they began rating them even higher and asking for them repeatedly. The lessons learned: Absence makes the heart grow fonder, and perhaps Eve was set up, baby.

Challenge #7

Ready, set … cheat! Today is your cheat day, but only if you really cleared out the fridge and pantry in Challenge #2. Otherwise, you'll need to read it again and earn a cheat day when another one comes around (and it will). Remember your two food demons? Pick one of them and enjoy!

Why It Works

Cutting out all carbs or sugar or fried foods forever is a sure setup for failure. Why? We're only human, and life is too short to completely deny yourself something you love. That said, the cheat day is the exception and not the rule.

Knowing that you get a cheat day every few days or so gives you a finish line and a reward. It breaks up a difficult week of being "good" into smaller increments so that the overall goal of eating well is achieved in the end. It also makes you appreciate the quality of your food even more. For example, on a cheat day, you won't settle for a bag of plain M&Ms anymore (even though you used to keep a one-pound bag in your desk to munch on throughout the workday). Nope. On a cheat day, only the finest Belgian chocolate Häagen-Dazs will do. Ahhh.

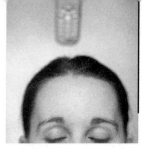

Day 8
Your Body
Is a Cell Phone

My cell phone company charges me almost $100 for about 500 minutes on my plan. I rarely use the thing and haven't moved forward at all with the technological advances in the category. In fact, my cell phone is so large and outdated at this point that it resembles the old Maxwell Smart shoe phone. My minutes don't roll over. I either use them or lose them. But I've bought them at a price, regardless. They're mine to squander if I choose.

In much the same way, I own my body, every precious nerve, muscle fiber, and blood vessel. I can do as I choose with this body, but there are consequences far greater than the overage charges of my cell phone.

Because of MS, I became a complete klutz, twisting ankles, tripping on stairs, knocking over glasses, and chipping plates. My answer to the dilemma: I signed up for basketball. I'm 5'3" and hadn't played the game since high school. Actually, I should clarify: I was on the team in high school, but I kept the bench warm. In the adult rec league I joined this year, my team was comprised of ex-college standouts. All of the women were taller, younger, and in better shape than me. None of them appeared to get confused and throw the ball to the opposite team. I joined because I needed to work on my stop-and-start speed and hand-eye coordination. A game provided a way for me to have fun while doing it. The result: I still suck at basketball, but I am quick and agile on my feet in a way I haven't been since my early twenties.

Challenge #8

Join up for basketball, soccer, tennis, racquetball, flag football, lacrosse, dance, or Ultimate Frisbee. Whether you join a class or a team, sign up today and work it into your schedule. It doesn't matter if you can make all the classes or not, even though you paid for them all. Like those cell phone minutes that don't roll over, you'll benefit from those that you use and perhaps become more committed to using them all because you've paid in advance. Your health is worth the entire cost.

Why It Works

Ball sports such as basketball, tennis, racquetball, and soccer provide stimulation for fast-twitch muscle fibers and enhance hand-eye coordination. As kids, we tore up the playgrounds with our quick stops, starts, and side-to-side motions. As adults, we rarely use those skills, and as a result, we're not as agile as we age. Muscles and nerves that aren't stimulated die slowly. The sports listed in the challenge above will bring you back to the playground, court, and gym.

Use it or lose it. We don't have to regress and become feeble and uncoordinated as we grow old. Choose to dance and play into your 80s and beyond. Can you hear me now?

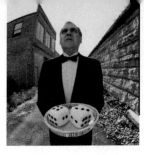

Day 9
Make Good Choices

Your stomach growls and you reach for a menu. You've never been so hungry. But when you look at the menu, the pages are blank. The waiter comes over with his hands behind his back. He extends his arms to you with both fists closed tightly. As he uncurls the fingers of the left hand, you see nine little foil-wrapped Hershey Kisses. In the right he has nothing, because he can't possibly hold all the food he's about to show you. He reaches behind him and presents you with a plate of herb-crusted Italian turkey meatloaf, a side of homemade applesauce, and a mixed-greens house salad with a light vinaigrette. You start to salivate.

"Choose," the waiter says. "Both meals have the same number of calories, but which will leave you more satisfied?" The waiter is a bit of a smart aleck, but he does have a point. If all menus were presented with two columns of food choices, containing a healthy meal on the right and an unhealthy meal on the left with identical calories, it would make our decisions so much easier, especially if both selections were tantalizing in their own way. But forget about the snappy waiter for now, because you are the food server in your own home. You decide which foods are available and presented, and you can decide how many calories they contain and whether or not you like them.

Challenge #9

Before you head to the store, list two fruits you really enjoy, two healthy snack items (yogurt, almonds, soy ice cream, energy bars, yogurt-covered raisins, honey-drizzled almonds), two healthy beverages (soy milk, fat-free milk, not-from-concentrate juices, natural sodas), two types of whole-grain bread (honey, wheat, multi-grain), two types of whole-grain, high-fiber cereal, two vegetables, two meats/meat substitutes, and so on. The idea is to have an arsenal of good foods you enjoy that are also healthy for you, ready to choose from as you shop.

Why It Works

The food industry is a marketing monster. I swear, blinking neon-lit packaging and chocolate-scented cardboard are next. They know what to do to get you to pick up their products and put them into your cart. Preparing a list of food items you really like eating that are also good for you will give you better choices when the Hershey Kiss foil, glinting in the fluorescent lighting, catches your eye.

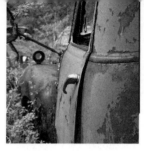

Day 10
Outrunning Trauma

There's a rusted red Ford truck that convalesces a few blocks from where I live. I run by this relic every day. At ten years old, I was abused in an identical truck. I can't believe they still run or that anyone would consider them a collector's item worth hanging on to … like an old 1965 Mustang or a 1975 Corvette. I can smell the interior of the truck a block away. See the dash. Feel the seat. It's that clear to me, and my heart races as fast as my feet as I go by. Still, I refuse to alter my route.

Abuse caused me to hide my body for years. I was in my twenties before I would even think of running in just my sports bra in the 100-degree Texas heat. At 105 pounds and 5'3", I'd buy a size large in shirts and jackets. I never realized what I was doing until a colleague of mine pointed it out while we were on a shopping spree. Perhaps my need to cover my body was a manifestation of guilt. Or maybe I wanted to appear bigger and more formidable. I'm thankful that my need to conceal the scars of abuse did not culminate into an eating disorder or the desire to hide myself in layers of fat instead of layers of clothing. But, like most of us, I did not emerge unscathed.

So why do I run by the Ford? Anything else might allow the truck to win. I am victorious over my past, and I won't allow anything or anyone who harmed me take away something I love so dearly now. I'm not speaking about the running here, though I really do love running. But more importantly, I love me. I deserve to be healthy in mind, body, and spirit. So I feel free, not bound, as I run by the rusted red truck. Each step reminds me that I am stronger than the past behind me.

Challenge #10

Take a moment to think about the biggest reason you have been unable or unwilling to embrace a healthy you. Write this down on a sheet of paper. Is it fear of failure? Low self-esteem from verbal abuse or neglect? Perhaps you give your best to everyone but yourself, or you do little things to sabotage your health as a manifestation of scars that people can't see. Take a moment to figure out where these roadblocks originated. Get to the root of your obsession with overeating, alcohol abuse, or neglecting yourself. You cannot rise up to be healthy if you are shackled to the ground with the wounds of your past. Consider making an appointment with a professional who can help you work through these issues.

Why It Works

Identifying those things that are holding you back from living a full life takes self-examination. Writing down those things that hinder you gives them a name and makes them a little less powerful. Awareness is the first step toward healing.

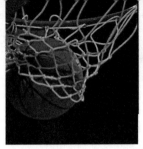

Day 11
Get By with a Little Help from Your Friends

You may not have heard of Jason McElwain. He doesn't play in a rock band or star in movies with Reese Witherspoon. He's not a Nobel-prize-winning physicist or Pulitzer-prize-winning author. But in 2006 he made history.

During his senior year, Jason was the manager for the basketball team at Greece Athena High School in Rochester, New York. Jason is autistic and had never gotten to play in a real game, but he still enjoyed being involved with the team.

In the very last game of the season, Jason's coach, Jim Johnson, added Jason to the roster and gave him a uniform. At the very least, he wanted Jason to be able to sit on the bench with the others.

With four minutes left in the game, Greece Athena led its opponent by double-digits, so Jim put Jason into the game. Jason's teammates welcomed the idea, as he had provided the spark of inspiration that had kept them victorious all season. If he stayed home sick for a day, they missed him. So the moment he stepped on the floor, they passed him the ball.

Jason's first shot missed the rim entirely. His teammates gave him the ball again. In front of a packed and cheering gym, he fumbled a layup right underneath the basket. He might have stopped right there, but his team and coach wouldn't give up on him. They passed him the ball yet a third time—and magic happened.

Over the next three minutes, Jason sunk six three-pointers in a row and made an additional two-point shot for a total of 20 points. At the end of the game, his team and his classmates carried him off the court on their shoulders.

Someone supporting and believing in you makes the impossible possible.

Challenge #11

Think of someone who will support you on this journey to good health. Who can you tell about the work you've been doing? Who will agree to be in your cheering section? Select this person and ask him or her to join you for a bike ride or walk after work or at lunch to tell him or her about your commitment.

Why It Works

We all need someone to believe in us when we're tackling the seemingly impossible. Telling someone your goals means that you become accountable not just to yourself but to the other person as well. Once it's out there, there's no taking it back. Let a friend or family member cheer you on to victory.

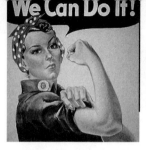

Day 12
The Do-It-Yourself Woman

In 2005 Ellen MacArthur became the first person to sail solo and nonstop around the world in the record time of 71 days, 14 hours, 18 minutes, and 33 seconds. She faced 65 mile-per-hour winds, brutal storms, a near-catastrophic accident with a whale, and loneliness.

Lynne Cox is the only person ever to swim 2.1 ice-water miles across the English Channel in a time of 9 hours and 36 minutes. Lynne says she swims because "It gives me a chance to explore the great waterways of the world."

Tiny Lynn Hill took on free-climbing the Nose of El Capitan in Yosemite in 1993 and repeated the route the following year. No other climber in the world has been able to duplicate her feat.

Ninety-year-old Jenny Wood-Allen recently completed the London Marathon, becoming the oldest woman to do so. She ran her very first marathon at age 71.

If you're seeing a pattern here, it's that women possess the power to do incredible things—not in spite of being women, perhaps because of it.

While we need to rely on others and be able to ask for help, it's also nice to know that we still have the capacity to handle all tasks, large and small. There's a confidence that only self-sufficiency brings. The women above believe and know that they can do anything they put their minds and bodies to. Likewise, there are no limits to the record-breaking feats or accomplishments you might achieve. Start with small steps, Superwoman, and you'll be on your way.

Challenge #12

No help today. Forget your assistant at work grabbing
something off the fax machine for you, your kids helping
with the dishes, your husband mowing the lawn or
unscrewing jars, and the bagger taking your groceries out
to your car. Today you will run back up the stairs for
something you forgot or go to FedEx to ship a package
rather than calling them to pick it up. Do your own
chores and run your own errands. You will become super-
human today.

Why It Works

Helen Reddy was the first to coin it: "I am woman; hear
me roar." Little did she know that the do-it-yourself
woman would also be burning about 150 calories more
than her couch-ridden counterparts. Today, the dishwasher.
Tomorrow, the world.

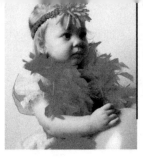

Day 13
See Yourself Beautiful

Nike, Dove, and Weight Watchers. What do these three companies have in common? All three have jumped on the hottest advertising trend to connect with female consumers—celebrate your body as it is, in all its various shapes and sizes. The underlying message: Hey, we get you. You're tired of being told you have to look like Uma Thurman to be considered beautiful.

This well-illustrated concept speaks volumes to me and to other women who have responded with a chorus of "It's about time!" One Nike ad presents us with a well-rounded hiney and the headline "My butt is shaped like the letter C." The next in the series gives us a pair of women's legs as big as Joe Montana's and the tagline "I have thunder thighs." Dove ads feature real women who are curvy and voluptuous in untouched photographs with the teaser "Let's face it, firming the thighs of a size 2 supermodel is no challenge." Meanwhile, Weight Watchers connects to us through a powerful television spot. Set to the Cher hit "Song for the Lonely," the ad shows women uniting in the struggle to lose weight and accepting themselves and each other in the process. These messages pack an emotional wallop. In fact, they reverberate down to my last few jiggly bits and parts. I am reminded that I am beautiful just as I am.

This message of self-acceptance sits at the heart of *Women's Adventure Magazine*. I created it because women seemed to have so few other media choices like it. As far as I know, we are the only active-women's magazine without a quick-fix, "thinner-thighs-in-thirty-days" focus.

I like to envision a world where women will kayak around a glacier shadowed by the wings of bald eagles soaring above them. They will climb the stairs of a lighthouse with a toddler in tow to marvel at the ocean from the top. They will walk an ancient trail to examine petroglyphs. And they will never once ask, "Does this make my butt look big?"

Challenge #13

Strip naked and walk to a full-length mirror. Start with your feet and end with your hair. Name one positive attribute for each body part. Try not to laugh or minimize the compliments or negate the power of what you have said with the word *but* afterwards. Listen and believe.

Why It Works

Accept your body. Know that you are beautiful inside and out. Hating our bodies is something reinforced by the media. You cannot become healthy if you are constantly at war with your self-image. Your stomach may have stretch marks, but maybe it created two unique individuals who may change the world (after they finish their juice, of course). Your hair may have more gray than you'd like, but each strand is soft and frames your face like a work of art. You are not your crummy job, the cellulite on your thighs, the dented fender in the garage, or the arthritis in your hands. You are beautiful.

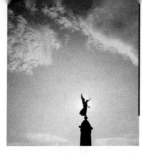

Day 14
Your One Unpredictable Life

In the '90s I worked for an athletic shoe company and traveled all over the United States signing athletes to endorsement contracts. As a 23-year-old woman, the job gave me the chance to see and experience our country in ways I would never have been able to afford otherwise. To prevent his staff from burning out, the CEO of our company extended every perk to us from first-class tickets to stays at the Ritz. Large expense accounts made young people more eager to travel and less grumpy about leaving friends and family behind. His bribery worked. While I often returned home exhausted and jet lagged, I knew I'd been blessed with a terrific opportunity. Before I turned 27, I had visited every state except for North Dakota, South Dakota, and Alaska.

On one of my trips to a remote part of New Mexico, I'd flown in late, grabbed a rental car, and headed out to find my hotel. The deserted street whispered a warning to me I couldn't quite identify. I just knew something wasn't right, the way a person knows it's about to rain or that the dinner rolls in the oven are about to burn. I stopped at a red light. Checked my map. Another car pulled up alongside me. I glanced over. The car was a late model Camry. The woman at the wheel smiled over at me. We sat. No cross traffic in sight. The red light stretched on, mocking us both.

As the light turned green, I pressed the accelerator. I'd no sooner gone five feet than a pickup truck blew its red light and slammed into the Camry, sending both vehicles, connected from the impact, skidding toward me. I swerved, honked, swore, and prayed until all motion stopped. I hadn't been hit.

I looked to my left. The Camry was crushed. The truck had hit the woman on the driver's side without ever braking. No one inside seemed to be moving. I started to open my door when I heard yelling from the truck. Two men ran from it toward my car. One carried a shotgun. The other, the one standing beside my window just two moments later, held a handgun pointed at my head. My car was still running. They wanted my car.

I blinked a couple of times before flooring the accelerator. At the next pay phone, I dialed 911.

Challenge #14

Life is short. Despite my best efforts to see the world and stay healthy, I could have been dead before my 24th birthday. As a friend of mine who survived breast cancer says, "Hey, none of us get out of this alive." If you knew you were dying tomorrow, you'd have that extra slice of chocolate cake and go skydiving. So, today is another Cheat Day! Remember your food vices. Pick one and go to town. You've earned it.

Why It Works

You could get hit by a bus tomorrow, so remember to wear clean underwear, but forget about wiping away the grease on your chin from the fried chicken. There's just not enough time.

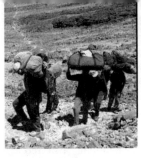

Day 15
Driven by Hunger

Droop-proof your butt. Ten-minute abs. Did you know they even have a pill you can take now called "Tasteless"? Take the pill and you won't be able to taste sugar anymore. That's right. Coke will taste just like plain soda water. Peanut M&Ms will just taste like peanuts. How can we live life to its fullest if we can no longer taste, touch, smell, or see it?

On a trip to Africa, I talked to our guides about their views of Americans. They love us for our tourism dollars but don't understand the concept of outdoor recreation. My guide up Kilimanjaro is named Jamaica. He's climbed the highest mountain on the continent more times than he can count. The average annual income for a Tanzanian is $200. Jamaica will make at least that much in tips from each member of our group on the seven-day trek. It's a classic catch-22. The erosion and devastation caused by tourism kills the mountain. Lack of tourism might kill the African economy.

Jamaica tells me, "Africans don't climb Kilimanjaro for fun. We climb it because it provides good jobs, and we must feed our families." I tell Jamaica, "Americans work long hours behind desks to feed their families. We no longer have to physically procure our food, clothing, and shelter. So, we are soft. We come to the mountain to test our strength and stamina." It seems a ludicrous explanation of our culture as I watch the porters pass us on the trail carrying at least 100 pounds of our team's gear per person. Some of the soles of their shoes are missing, and they layer their cotton or nylon clothing for warmth. They don't have sub-zero rated sleeping bags or Gore-Tex hiking boots or 800-down-filled jackets. The porters and guides are amazing athletes. But they do not hunger for medals or trophies. They just hunger, and their hunger drives them onward despite adversity.

As Americans, we try to quell our hunger and stifle our cravings instead of letting our hunger drive us forward. There are no quick fixes. There is no easy route up the mountain. No porters to carry you and your bags, and that includes the makers of fen-phen and sugar substitutes. If you had to climb the mountain in order to live, you would let nothing stand in your way. And so now I will tell you the absolute truth: you must climb the mountain in order to live.

Challenge #15

Take the longest distance you've run or walked, ever, and double it. Today is the day you surpass your expectations. Redefine the impossible.

Why It Works

The distance today is what is important, not how you achieve it. Walk, stroll, run, sprint, jog, or do laps at the mall, but double your farthest distance. If you need to stop and rest, it's okay. You will burn the same amount of calories whether you walk, run, or crawl. Though the intensity and the type of activity you choose may have other benefits (cardiovascular and muscular), the caloric burn remains the same. Climb the mountain at any pace you wish, but don't stop until you touch the summit.

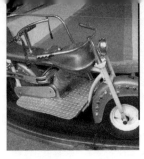

Day 16
You Rascal, You

Walt Disney World is home to more rides than just the Tower of Terror and Pirates of the Caribbean. It's hard to take a single step without first checking your blind spot for motorized Rascal scooters that might roar past and run you over. There's nothing wrong at all with assisted transportation. If and when I need a little help getting around, I plan on painting my Rascal purple and putting streamers on the handlebars. But seeing so many scooters and wheelchairs in one place made me wonder if all of the people in them really needed the extra lift. Could these items meant to help us out become instead a self-fulfilling prophecy? If I get good at sleeping late, letting someone else carry my groceries, or riding in a wheelchair, I just may perfect the art of it. Truth be told, I don't want to get good at not walking or carrying my own produce. I'd guess that no one does. But the more we allow someone or something else to do the day-to-day for us, the less able our body will become at doing those things. Soon we won't have the choice. Our bodies will get too good at resting. They'll become the Olympians of sitting and riding, and we'll become passive passengers in the life we've created.

Shortcuts are easy, but in the long run, they rob us of our independence. Whether you realize it or not, each day you're training your body for life. Don't take shortcuts until you have to.

Challenge #16

Take a moment to think about how you spend your day. What shortcuts are you taking in your life that may be hurting you? We talked on Day 12 about the extra calories burned and the confidence built from handling your own chores. But we didn't discuss the use-it-or-lose-it philosophy as it applies to chores. While no one thinks they'll miss stretching to grab a plate off the highest shelf or washing the car or plowing the driveway, it's a sad day when those things are no longer possible, because it means we've lost our independence. And that's a precious gift.

If you spend ten years of your life steadily allowing others to do things for you and you suddenly end up alone, will you still have enough strength in your hands to turn the doorknob or lift a gallon of milk? Today you will pretend that you are completely on your own. Cancel your housecleaner or the boy who mows your lawn. Don't order takeout. Savor the fact that you can still do things on your own. Enjoy each movement.

Why It Works

You're too young for assisted living. Start viewing your body as your greatest tool for success in life. Keep it in shape and able to do the basic activities of daily life. If you try to open a jar three times and fail, your three tries will have been great physical therapy. The more you give up, the more that function will be gone for good. Fight for your health—especially on the days when you may find it easier to give up.

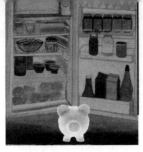

Day 17
Serving It Up

If you've ever seen a golden retriever eat, you know
that they just can't stop until the bowl is empty. Labs
and goldens can clear a plate so fast that they are actually
at risk for having their stomachs flip over, a dangerous
condition that can lead to death. My Shiba Inu, Biscuit,
throws up every time she eats beef because she's allergic.
Still, if I held out a juicy steak, she'd gnaw off my hand to
get to it. Doesn't she know better? Is it selective memory or
instinct? Lack of intelligence or basic survival? Why would
she eat something she knows will make her sick?

Before I start feeling superior over my canine buddies, I'll have to fess up to scarfing down an entire pint
of Ben & Jerry's New York Super Fudge Chunk and
drinking half a bottle of Merlot last night. I started, and
I couldn't stop. Once I'd had a bite or two of the ice
cream, I figured I might as well go all the way. Same with
the wine. One glass turned to three and before I knew it,
I was toasting Richard Simmons and Jenny Craig for their
iron will and discipline.

To assuage my guilt, I write and rewrite the rules
around the cravings. I justify. I swear on my bean sprouts
it won't happen again. And it doesn't, for a while. It's the
"for a while" part I learn to celebrate. The limits I've set
down work 75 percent of the time, and rather than beat
myself up over the quite piggish 25 percent, I've learned
to be proud of the restraint I've acquired against my
nature, instinct, and the basic need we all have as humans
to finish an entire pint of Ben & Jerry's in one sitting.

Challenge #17

What's a serving size? Today you will read the packaging on everything you eat. In fact, don't eat anything today that doesn't have a label, just so you can enjoy the experiment. At the top left of each label, the food manufacturer defines the serving size. For example, a jar of mixed nuts lists a serving size as approximately 27 pieces. Then, as you read on, you'll see that they tell you how many calories, fat, and sodium can be found in that single serving.

For example, the label on an 11.5-ounce container of mixed nuts tells us that a single serving will supply 170 calories. Not too bad for a snack, considering 27 nuts would be more than filling. So today, eat a single serving size or less of your meals and snacks and stop there.

Why It Works

If you're not paying attention, you'll sit at your desk with that same little tin of mixed nuts mentioned above and eat until it echoes. The damage? Let's say a normal human being watching their weight should eat around 1,500 to 2,000 calories per day. According to the label, that tin of nuts holds 12 servings at 170 calories per serving. Eat the whole can and you've just consumed 2,040 calories before you've had lunch or dinner (and by the way, 1,500 of those calories came from fat).

So, while serving sizes may seem ridiculous and random at times (I've read that 3/4 of a spear of a pickle equals one serving and that a personal pan pizza serves two), they help us pay attention and set limits, something our canine buddies can only rely on us to do for them.

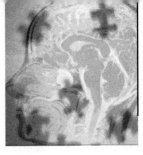

Day 18
Life's a Puzzle

"Count back from 100, subtracting by seven." My neurologist scribbles on a pad of paper. He looks away as I try to mimic Dustin Hoffman in the movie *Rain Man*. I wish he'd laugh to cut the tension. I've disclosed to him that I'm having a hard time finding the right word lately. I forget letters and have to go back and correct my work. I'm misspelling words and unable to recall others. Words have become like old relatives I recognize as familiar but can't seem to place into the family tree. I explain to Dr. Pratt that I'm a writer. I make my living with words. Confusing the usage of *are* and *our* is unacceptable in my line of work. And scary. I'm scared.

I count back from 100 and take my time. I mumble, "93, 86, 79, 73, 67, 60." I wring my hands because I know I'm making mistakes. Not in my math. My math is perfect. But I've forgotten whether I'm supposed to be subtracting by seven or by six and am alternating between the two.

The fact that I know what is causing my mental collapse is no more comforting than knowing the answer to whether the potato salad you ate at the barbecue has been left out too long. You sense impending doom. My MS has caused scarring in the parietal and temporal lobes of my brain. The brain is a giant puzzle with pieces designed to handle various tasks. The left parietal lobe handles writing, language, and mathematics. The frontal lobe is the emotional control center of the brain and is the most often injured because it sits behind the forehead.

It directs our fine-motor skills, sex drive, spontaneity, facial expression, and spatial relationships. The occipital lobes, at the back of the skull, handle vision and visual perception. The temporal lobes are associated with memory, word recognition and placement, personality, music, and recall. They sit below the frontal lobes and in front of the occipital lobes. Finally, the cerebellum, at the base of the skull, controls voluntary movement, balance, and muscle tone. Left and right sides of lobes in each section of the brain often handle different things. Every piece of the puzzle is important. Lose a piece, and you're left with a giant hole to fill and a picture that no longer makes sense. Save and protect each critical piece, and you'll become and remain a complete picture of health.

The normal aging process does its damage on our brains in much the same way it affects our bodies. Brain activity grows slower with time. How slow may depend on the effort you expend trying to work out your mind as much as your body.

Challenge #18

Grab the daily newspaper and turn to the crossword puzzle. Sit down and work it. If you don't finish in one sitting, save it for later and continue to come back to it throughout the day. If you are already a crossword hound, then add a different puzzle to the one you already do. For example, the Cryptoquote, Jumble, or Suduko. You can also try games such as Scrabble, Boggle, and Trivial Pursuit with your family and friends.

Why It Works

Mental gymnastics will keep your mind agile and flexible for years to come.

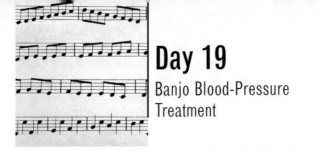

Day 19
Banjo Blood-Pressure Treatment

In 1976, during his *Saturday Night Live* monologue, Steve Martin said, "You just can't sing a depressing song when you're playing the banjo." He went on to try, and of course, it just can't be done. The banjo is just a happy instrument. We tend to think that in order to improve our health and well-being, we must make drastic and difficult changes in our lives. For the most part, that theory holds true. However, there are small, easy, fun things we could incorporate into our lives that have been scientifically proven to boost our health, such as:

1. Petting a puppy lowers blood pressure.
2. Watching fish swim lowers stress more than most types of meditation.
3. Singing a happy song makes you smile.
4. Getting a few minutes of natural sun (or buying a light box) elevates the depression-busting endorphin and seratonin levels in your body.
5. Smiling, whether or not you mean it, lifts the fog of a bad mood and makes you start to feel happier.
6. Laughing at a 30-minute sitcom or a favorite comedy film eases muscle tension, lowers blood pressure, strengthens the immune system, reduces stress-hormone production, increases your ability to handle pain, and gives your lungs and abs an aerobic workout.

But then, you always knew laughter was the best medicine.

Challenge #19

Add something new to your life today. If you've been thinking about adopting a cat or dog from the local humane society, it's the perfect time to sign the papers. If that's too much of a commitment, try getting a colorful Siamese fighting fish and placing him in a small bowl on your desk at work. Or you can take in the latest flick from Ben Stiller or Adam Sandler tonight. Just choose one of the above, relax, and be happy.

Why It Works

Scientific studies show that laughter, prayer, pets, meditation, massage, sunlight, singing, and fish tanks benefit our emotional and physical health. You may not enjoy running or taking your blood-pressure pills, but what's not to like about a good banjo-pickin' song or a warm puppy? Change your natural environment to make your life better.

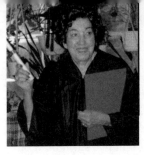

Day 20
It's Never Too Late for Adventure

Frances Theall graduated from Sam Houston State University with a bachelor of fine arts in 1988, a year ahead of me. She lived in the dorm and commuted home in her red Mustang on the weekends. With two boyfriends, one in-state and one out, she knew how to get attention from the opposite sex. This might be the typical college co-ed story, except that the student I'm talking about was my 82-year-old grandmother.

My grandmother's home in Texas sported the requisite doily-covered couches and floral-patterned walls, but the stereotypes ended there. Her original artwork hung in every room, and the paintings spoke of a life much too big to capture with oil strokes on canvas. In her photo albums, she sits astride a camel in Egypt and stands along the Great Wall of China. She drinks wine in a gondola and flirts with a hand on the shoulder of the gondolier. She sports a beret in Paris and dances through a crowd in Spain. The photos appear barely able to stop her from motion. She winks, head tilting back with laughter, moving out of the frame.

When I was 22, she took me on a trip to see Europe. It was her fourth. In London, Paris, and Rome, I etched my grandmother's history into my memory, alongside the dates of buildings in the ancient cities we toured. These are the things I remember. Frances walked every day of her life. In hotels or bad weather, she'd walk laps around the room itself for 30 minutes. She carried a flask filled with whiskey and swore by it when traveling. A

100-proof shot of liquor killed any bugs in the food or water that might make her ill while jaunting internationally. She'd lost most of her hair by her early 80s and wore a wig to stay youthful looking. Underneath the wig she dyed each remaining strand jet black, just in case. In her 90s she could sometimes be caught sneaking up on the roof to sweep off pine needles and toss down dead branches.

Until the day that she died, she painted, took Spanish lessons, and headed the local garden club. Never once in all the time I was fortunate enough to know her did I ever hear her say, "I'm too old to do that now." Anyone saying otherwise only provided the challenge she needed to prove them wrong.

Challenge #20

You are never too old for a new adventure. Today you will pick an adventurous pursuit and do it. Bungee jumping, rock climbing, paintball, paragliding, backpacking, skiing, and mountain biking might be a few ideas. Choose an adventure and participate in it today. If you don't have access to the above, then try a new location for your typical workout. Drive to the zoo or botanical gardens for your daily walk or run. Bike alongside a lake or climb a tree. Just get creative, get outside, and Adventurcise.

Why It Works

Your mind and body need a jump start from the boring humdrum of everyday life. Trying new things and continually learning keeps us young in mind, body, and spirit. Heading outdoors, regardless of the weather, exposes us to the beauty of the world around us. We live in a tremendously beautiful and mysterious place, and our greatest regret may be that we lack enough time on this earth to explore every single inch of it.

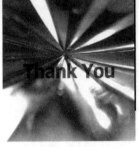
Thank You

Day 21
Power of
Positive Thinking

Read the following words: fool, ugly, inept, stupid. How did you feel when you were reading each word? Now read the following: beautiful, wise, strong, worthy, capable. How did you feel this time? Words hold the power to affect human beings in profound ways. Some say the energy of words causes transformation that can be scientifically proven. Psychologists have spoken for decades about self-fulfilling prophecy, theologians tout the power of prayer, and parenting experts warn us to be careful about the lasting impact of negative words on our children.

More recently, a man named Dr. Masaru Emoto tested the power of words on water crystallization. He taped words including *thank you* and *fool* on separate bottles of water and then froze the bottles. The bottles with positive words formed exceptionally beautiful crystals. Those with negative words formed no crystals or clusters. He tried the experiment in other languages with similar results. Knowing that human beings are predominantly made of water and that the universe requires it for the existence of life, we might deduce that words alone have the power to heal or destroy us.

Whether you believe in Dr. Emoto's experiment or write him off as a quack, you'll find that the words you hear and say affect how you feel about yourself and those around you. Which, to say the least, is most powerful in itself.

Challenge #21

Cheat Day! Today pick one of your two food vices you swore off in Challenge #2 and enjoy. Instead of feeling guilty, tell yourself with each bite how much you deserve this treat. Praise yourself for being so strong. Pat yourself on the back. Tell yourself that you have earned this reward because you are committed, disciplined, capable, and confident. While you're at it, you may want to add a day at the spa just to make sure the message of love to yourself gets through.

Why It Works

Babies who aren't held or told they are loved end up with certain parts of their brains forever inactivated. As adults, we have a voice. Speak up. Tell yourself what you need to hear to be healthy, happy, and to continue to grow.

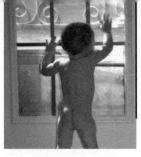

Day 22
One Precious Life

Sharon White is 39. She owns her own business. Tells it like it is. Takes in all strays, both furry and human, because her heart is too big not to. Back pain brings her to the doctor. Ovarian cancer leaves her bald and skinny. Her 40th-birthday roast is standing-room-only. Over lunch she tells me that her cancer is a gift. She is not supposed to live. Her treatments have not worked. "I get to know," she says. "Everyone's time is short, but I know it in a real way. Do I want to die? No. But we're all going to. My cancer is a gift. It's a wake-up call to live life to its fullest. Some people don't get that wake-up call. They miss out."

Sharon has altered quite a few things in her life since the diagnosis. She rarely drinks and has banished refined sugar from her diet. She's more active, and she travels everywhere. In addition, she ended an energy-draining relationship, even though she dreaded fighting cancer without a significant other. She found out who she could lean on and considered this new revelation another treasure. Her idea is to truly live her life fully, and it surprises her when she sees other healthy people squandering it.

"I have a friend who is always depressed, always negative. She doesn't seem to enjoy life at all," Sharon says. "She might live to be 100, but I wouldn't trade the hand I've been dealt with hers at any price. Who wants to live 100 miserable years? Talk about a death sentence."

Challenge #22

You've been given one precious life. Write down five
things you'd like to do or see before your time on this
earth is up. Try not to censor your thoughts. Think big.
Review the list. Pick one of those things and schedule it
on your calendar this year.

Why It Works

We seem to find the time and money for those things that
are most important to us. Today you are moving yourself
to the top of that list. Regret, guilt, stress, and boredom
all negatively affect your health and rub off on those you
love. Live life to its fullest, and you'll have more positive
energy to give to those around you and more creativity at
work and home.

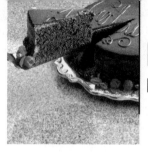

Day 23
Eat Me

Remember *Alice in Wonderland*? I like to think that supplements are like the cake with currants on top that Alice ate. Eat me. Poof! Instant results. Of course, the results weren't exactly as she'd hoped.

Research is important. While the Food and Drug Administration doesn't regulate supplements, they've been known to help individuals in a variety of ways. For me, magnesium/calcium supplements at a 2:1 ratio eased my muscle soreness and cramping after a hard workout. I wasn't getting enough magnesium or my body wasn't readily absorbing it. Either way the supplements made a huge change in my life and my ability to recover from even the most basic exercises.

It's always preferable to change your diet and get nutrients through the foods you consume, but it's not always easy or practical. The nutrient quality of our food declines more every year. Eating organic helps, but it's still not the ultimate solution. If you're missing basic nutrients in the foods you eat, your body will tell you. Listen to it, or, for a more complete picture, get tested by a holistic practitioner. Basic and painless diagnostic tests can tell you what your body needs.

Challenge #23

Think about your body for a moment. Are you always low on energy? Do you get frequent muscle cramps and spasms? Is your complexion a mess? Do you suffer from joint stiffness? How's your immune system? Take a look at www.wholefoods.com and www.wildoats.com and review their handy information on supplements and nutrition. Then head to your local organic store and let the magic begin.

Why It Works

As hard as we try, it's difficult to eat right. Each person has different physical needs anyway, and not everyone will thrive on the new food pyramid. You are unique. Figure out what your body needs and be ready to supplement it, if necessary, with the right vitamin or mineral. Start today.

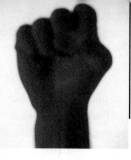

Day 24
Don't Just Do It for Yourself

Whether or not you realize it, your efforts at improving your health will have an impact beyond you. Consider Ellen Johnson-Sirleaf, a 67-year-old grandmother. She wears colorful clothing and crisp white pearls. But this year, Ellen Johnson-Sirleaf became the first female elected official in African history. Garnering an unprecedented 60 percent of the vote, Ellen sits as the president of Liberia, an African nation plagued by civil unrest, corruption, illiteracy, and an AIDS epidemic. But the impact she's had on women in the country shines a bright light on the possibilities for all Africans. After receiving a Harvard education and being able to enjoy some of the immense opportunities of the West, she chose to return to Liberia to help it heal.

As the leader of an African nation, Ellen pushes tirelessly for women's rights to make certain rapists get prosecuted and women are hired for government positions, even looking toward setting hiring quotas. As she recently said to a *Newsweek* reporter, "Women know not only that they can compete, but also that they can excel. They can be mothers and also professionals. They know that we don't have to be stuck in the backyard."

Women know this, because they watched Ellen do the unthinkable—rise to power in Africa. Ellen Johnson-Sirleaf sets the bar to a higher place. Because of her example, Liberians can envision a healthy and strong nation as a possibility, not an unattainable dream.

Challenge #24

No matter where you are in your life, you are being watched by those around you. You are an example of success, and your health is no exception. Think about your family and your circle of friends today. As hard as it's been for you to walk down this path, there's someone else who views your efforts as inspirational. Find that person today, and have them join you for a 20-minute walk to catch up on life. Choose a pace where you are both able to talk without having to stop. You can go through a mall, the neighborhood, your building at work, or hop on the treadmills at a local fitness center. Let this person know about the changes you've been making and that today you were asked to have someone join you on your daily challenge.

Why It Works

You don't have to be a fitness instructor or wear a size-two dress to be a healthy example for those around you. The fact that you are taking active steps to improve your health is inspirational and admirable. People who know you and haven't made their own conscious decision yet to begin a health and fitness program are watching you. You are a mentor whether you've realized it or not. Your success tells those around you that it can be done. Regardless of how you feel from day to day, stick with it. Someone is always counting on you, and when you dig a little deeper, your courage will provide the inspiration they need to make a stand.

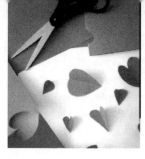

Day 25
What! No Seat Belts?

Rewind to the late 1960s. I'm four or five years old. The Beatles belt out "Michelle, my belle," and my parents play Twister in the living room. Dad has muttonchops, Mom a beehive. I sleep in bobby pins meant to curl my hair and don't manage to swallow or choke on any of them. There are no warnings on toys or plastic bags or sleds. I ride my bike without a helmet, get spanked at school, drink sodas, take aspirin, sleep on my stomach, back, and sides as an infant, and breathe in secondhand smoke. Before I am born, my mother chain-smokes, drinks alcohol moderately, eats as many heavily processed and chemically injected foods as she craves, and starts her day with a couple cups of coffee. Seat belts and car seats don't exist. I ride in the back of my grandfather's pickup truck with my cousins, and we stand up and wave at people on the sidewalks as we pass. My friends play kickball in the middle of the street and simply yell, "Car" if someone comes around the corner. Electrical outlets have no protective covers, cleaning products are stored under the kitchen sink without any locks, and childproof caps for drugs haven't been invented. Antibacterial soap, flu shots, and MRIs don't exist. My elementary school is made of asbestos and lead paint. Yet, miraculously, I survive.

Fast-forward to the present. The average human life span is around 82 years, versus 75 years in the 1960s. The difference is that we know more now. We make choices based on this knowledge. Granted, sometimes the information we receive seems as random as if the data resulted from a drunken dart game between scientists. It's not always easy to know what to believe and adopt into our lives. Mix together science, human examples of success, and a dose of common sense, though, and you've got a good recipe for longevity.

Challenge #25

Get educated about organics and whole foods today, because even these require updated knowledge in order to make the right decisions. Review the chart on page 54 and head to the grocery store. Try to purchase organic foods whenever possible and avoid highly processed foods, those with lots of chemicals, trans fats, dyes, and hydrogenated or partially hydrogenated oils. Choose to cook your own meals instead of heating up prepackaged and well-preserved ones. Go for fresh fruits and vegetables instead of canned and frozen, and avoid overcooking them, so they retain more nutrients. You are what you eat.

Why It Works

We're not living in caves or reading by oil lamps anymore. We've got centuries of research available to guide us to healthy and longer lives. Ignoring what's out there now would be, well, a little like riding a bike with no hands or helmet down a busy street.

Label	Where You See It	What You Think It Means
USDA Organic	produce, meat, poultry, packaged foods, beverages	Produce is grown without synthetic fertilizers, chemicals, sewage sludge, or genetic engineering. Organic animals are fed 100% organic feed that doesn't contain animal byproducts or growth hormones, and they have access to the outdoors.
Natural	on almost any food product	There is no artificial flavoring, coloring, preservatives, or artificial ingredients.
Free-Range	poultry, beef, eggs	The animal has lived a carefree life unconfined and outside.
Grass-Fed, Grain-Fed, or Pasture-Raised	meat, poultry	The animal has feasted on grass or grain or has spent its days grazing in a pasture.
No Hormones Added, No Hormones Administered	milk, yogurt, meat, poultry	The animal has had no added hormones during its lifetime.

What It Really Means

What to Look for Instead

Exactly that. All foods labeled "USDA Organic" must be verified as meeting the rigorous requirements set by the United States Department of Agriculture (USDA).

Though the USDA has set the official definition for "Natural" used on meat and poultry, the only ones regulating the claims on any product labeled as such are the ones manufacturing or marketing it. This term is meaningless.

USDA Organic

"Free-Range" is regulated only for poultry (not eggs), and the only requirement is that they have access to the outdoors—but for no specified amount of time; it could be five minutes. There is no regulation for the use of this label on beef.

Cage-Free. Although it doesn't tell how much space the animal has, it does tell you that it has been kept outside of a cage. Though it's not a regulated claim, many products that use this term give information on the labels.

There are no regulations for what an animal's diet actually comprises or for how much time is spent grazing in a pasture.

100% Grass- or Grain-Fed implies that the animal's diet was not supplemented with fillers. "Pasture-Finished" means that the animal spent most of its life in a field and wasn't sent to a feedlot to be fattened up. Again, not regulated, but ask your butcher about the producer.

The USDA already prohibits the use of hormones in hogs and poultry, so products carrying this label simply indicate guidelines that are already in place. Beef can be raised using hormones, so beef carrying this label can be significant. Once again, no regulations are in place, so ask your butcher about the producer.

Because many animal products contain traces of natural hormones, many manufacturers are turning to the term "No Hormones Added," especially on dairy products. And when used on things labeled "Organic," it is regulated.

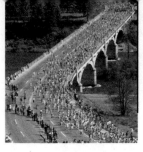

Day 26
Give and Get

If you've been to a Race for the Cure event benefiting breast cancer research, you've felt the unifying energy of the people there. Mostly women, including many breast cancer survivors and those who love them, walk and run a course marked out for them. Survivors wear pink hats. A few runners pin signs to their backs to signify they are walking in memory of someone who has died from the disease. Others wear signs showing their support of someone currently battling the disease. The women who surprise and inspire me the most are those who march with bald heads, appearing brave and frail at the same time.

I do not have breast cancer, and no one close to me has fought this disease. But with each step I take at the event, I feel I am doing something to help. Walking and running do more than strengthen me on that day, they show others they are not alone. The physical effort raises money. The solidarity and sheer mass numbers at these events (60,000 at the Denver Race for the Cure) give hope that a cure is close. And, while over 1 million people are expected to participate in a Komen Race for the Cure this year, it's clear that each individual makes a difference.

Challenge #26

Look up an event (race, walk, snowshoe, hike) taking place in your city within the next 30 days and sign up today. Race for the Cure events can be found listed at www.raceforthecure.org. Take a training walk or run at half the distance of the event today.

Why It Works

Surrounding yourself with those whose problems and losses may be greater than your own redirects your attention outward. It's hard to worry about how tired you feel on mile number two when the woman in front of you is in the middle of chemotherapy. Plus, the sheer energy of mass movement will carry you along to the finish. You will give others hope just by moving your feet.

Day 27
Toxic People

We can't control other people's actions, but we can control our reaction to them. My best friend, Jackie, learned this lesson the hard way. On the brink of bankruptcy, struggling with her health and her career, she joined her mom, dad, brother, sister-in-law, and two nephews on a family vacation to California. Jackie's mom is in her 60s now, but she's always been a "toxic person," directing sporadic fits of rage at friends, family, and even strangers.

This trip to California tested Jackie's mental and physical health. Stress was something she'd worked to alleviate from her life. A year before, she'd been diagnosed with high blood pressure. On this particular vacation, Jackie realized that she might need to alleviate contact with her own mother in order to protect her sanity and keep from ending up in the hospital with a stroke.

Within the first three days of the trip, Jackie's mom caused a scene at a local restaurant, the fitness center, and the golf course. She launched a grenade of words at anyone in her path, including her beloved family. At some point she collapsed into tears in the bedroom of the hotel suite. An hour later she emerged revived and ready to go do something fun. She issued no explanations or apologies. And when she asked Jackie, "Are we friends again?" Jackie answered, "Yes, but I have more things to be stressed about right now than whether or not housekeeping has given us enough hand towels."

Jackie's body took all the stress of those days and responded accordingly. Her head pounded with a migraine for two days. Her breath shortened into pants. She skipped a period altogether. When she returned home to Boston, she wrote a long letter to her mom, essentially telling her that she loved her but not her behavior. She asked that her mother see a counselor about her rage and the sense of entitlement that seemed to fuel it and that she get on some type of medication to even out these episodes. She let her mother know that she was free to ignore her daughter, but that based on that response, Jackie would choose whether or not to spend time with her. In setting up boundaries, Jackie protected her health.

Challenge #27

It's time to take inventory. Think about those closest to you—family, friends, neighbors, and coworkers. Which relationships contain unhealthy patterns of interaction? Are there toxic people you allow into your life? Take some time to identify your role and feelings with these people in various situations. What can you do to make things better? What healthy boundaries can you set up to protect yourself from further damage? Make those boundaries known by letter or conversation today.

Why It Works

Your health is much more than the physical state of your body. While you can't touch, taste, smell, or hear stress, it is the number one culprit behind illness and disease. If you want to live a longer life, you'll stop putting yourself into situations that cause unnecessary and preventable stress. You deserve to be loved and protected.

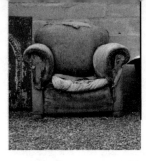

Day 28
Feed Your Surroundings to Feed Your Soul

Xorin Balbes, renowned home designer, restored the architecturally significant Lloyd Wright Sowden House and the Los Feliz replica of a 17th-century Italian villa. His client list includes high-profile celebrities from Broadway, film, and music. His gentle nature surprises those who meet him, and his home reflects a spiritual side. Xorin teaches his clients how to create an environment that will feed their creativity and spirit. He believes that the space around you feeds you whether you are aware of it or not. For example, the old ratty chair in the corner of your home reminds you that you are struggling with finances and can't afford a new one. It sends you that negative message every time you walk by it. It would be better for the space to be empty. Then you'd be thinking ahead to the endless possibilities. Objects hold power over us, which is different from materialism. The monetary value isn't important; the emotional impact is.

Restaurant owners also know this to be true as it relates to the color of a room. Oranges and reds cause people to eat faster. More turnover means more revenue. While you probably won't be going into fast food restaurants after reading this book, most of them use this color palette.

Smells evoke memory. A warm fire can make you think of snuggling under a blanket with someone you love. Vanilla might remind you of cookies baking in your grandmother's kitchen. This aroma alone may make you smile or feel warmth. That easily, your emotions respond to your environment. And, unlike most things in life, you can actually control what appears in the space around you. This has never been more important than now, when you are becoming the new and improved you.

Challenge #28

Take a moment to picture yourself a year from now. Who do you want to become? What will you look like? How will you feel about yourself, your body, your health? Now walk through your home. Would this new person you're becoming have just one mirror in her home? Would she play music and take bubble baths? Would her house have more natural sunlight? Go through your home. Open the drapes. Buy vanilla candles. Move your desk so that it faces out toward a view. Put up photos of people who inspire and believe in you. Post your walkathon race bib on the fridge. Make your kitchen an inviting place to cook healthy food. Change your home to reflect and draw out the best new you.

Why It Works

Your home speaks to you every day through the objects placed in it and by its sights, sounds, smells, and textures. If you live in a toxic environment, you'll receive unhealthy messages. Change your home or office to reflect the new you, and before you know it, she'll be there.

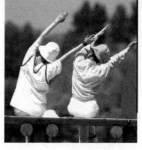

Day 29
Bend, Don't Break

Webster's Dictionary defines the word *core* this way: "the central or innermost part of anything; the most important part; essence; pith." The core of a tree allows it grow out in circles year after year as it climbs upward. It's this same core that flexes in the wind so that the tree bends rather than snapping in two. The tree stands strong because its core is dynamic, resilient, and adaptable.

If you think about human beings, you might make a literal definition of a person's core as their trunk, or stomach and abdominal muscles. A strong core protects the organs and delicate systems running inside of it. If your core is solid yet flexible, it can handle a punch to the gut and return to its original state. If it's flabby and soft, a tiny blow might level you.

If you speak in broader terms, you might define the core as the heart and soul of a person.

It has taken flexibility to get to this point in the book—a willingness at your core to adapt and change. Like the tree, you've learned to bend rather than break. In more physical terms, you've stretched the boundaries of what you thought might be possible and have grown stronger because of it. Your core has grown, but it didn't happen by accident. You chose to grow and expended the effort. The stretching made you stronger.

Challenge #29

Head to a yoga class today (most allow drop-ins and the cost is minimal). Yoga focuses on building core strength physically and mentally. Exercise is more than aerobic movement. Strength encompasses more than muscle mass. Yoga brings movement together with balance and strength for the ultimate workout of your mind, body, and soul.

Why It Works

Yoga connects your mind and body through slow, thoughtful movements. Knowing what your body can do will make you confident and determined, even when you are at rest. You will know that you can weather any storm.

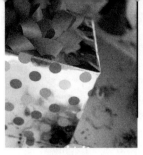

Day 30
Celebrate

Your good health is a lifelong commitment. Hopefully some of the exercises in this book challenged you to think about your mind, body, and spirit in new ways. The next step is to begin incorporating these lessons into your daily, weekly, and monthly routine. You might want to reread the book, and each day, try to extend the daily lesson into the entire week. On the third read, take each lesson and expand it through two weeks, and so forth, until the tips above become a normal part of your life.

Remember always that you are worth every effort and every ounce of dedication. You're alive, and that's something you'd like to continue. So embrace those things within your control that will make your life happier and healthier. You're on the road to feeling and looking great!

Challenge #30
Celebrate! You've made it through the end of this book and have taken an important 30 steps to better health. This deserves notice and reward. Call friends, toast with a glass of wine, or treat yourself to a day at the spa. Whatever you do, you've earned it.

Why It Works
No matter how you fared throughout this book, you read it from beginning to end and made an effort to complete each challenge. You may have accomplished a goal or made it to your own personal best. Either way, you've accomplished something grand and can be proud.

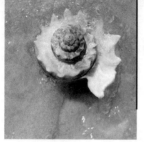

Sources

The author wishes to acknowledge the following source for material in the entry for Day 6:

Wansink, B., J. E. Painter, and J. North. "Bottomless Bowls: Why Visual Cues of Portion Size May Influence Intake." *Obesity Research* 13, no. 1 (January 2005): 93–100.

The author wishes to acknowledge the following sources for material in the entry for Day 19:

Becker, Marty. "Fish Help Humans Handle Stress." *Knight Ridder Tribune*, 14 September 2005.

Katcher, Aaron Honori. *New Perspectives on Our Lives with Companion Animals.* Philadelphia: Univ. of Pennsylvania Press, 1983.

McGhee, Paul. "Humor and Laughter Strengthen Your Immune System." *Newsletter* (January 2000), http://www.humor.ch/mcghee/mcghee_00_02.htm (accessed February 20, 2005).

Seaward, B. L. "Humor's Healing Potential." *Health Progress* 73, no. 3 (April 1992): 66–70.

Stuber, Margaret. "RX Laughter: A Study Designed to Understand the Biological Links between Humor and Laughing and Illness and Health in Children." Pediatric Chronic Pain Program, Los Angeles: UCLA, 2000, http://www2.health care.ucla.edu/pedspain/rp11_rxlaughter.htm (accessed February 26, 2005).

Wehr, Thomas A.; Duncan Jr., Wallace C.; Sher, Leo; Aeschbach, Daniel; Schwartz, Paul J.; Turner, Erick H.; Postolache, Teodor T.; and Norman E. Rosenthal. "A Circadian Signal of Change of Season in Patients with Seasonal Affective Disorder." *General Psychiatry* 58 (December 2001): 1108–1114.

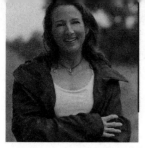

About the Author

Michelle Theall found out she had MS in 2003, just as she was putting the first issue of *Women's Adventure* magazine on press. As a former collegiate track athlete with a career built around fitness and health, Theall wondered if anyone would take her seriously now that she had a disease. Turns out, her readers were ready to have someone speak to them about health issues who was actually in the trenches working hard to live life to its fullest. Like many of her readers, Theall has a full-time job, a home to run, bills to pay, and no time or money for a personal trainer or in-home chef to prepare healthy meals.

A native Texan, Theall moved to Colorado 12 years ago to begin working in publishing with *Women's Sports + Fitness* magazine in Boulder. In 1998 she started her own media company, Teal Mountain Media Group, to work with niche magazines, Web sites, and manufacturers in the sports industry. She continues to publish *Women's Adventure* magazine (www.womensadventuremagazine.com) as the only women-specific outdoor sports title on the planet and remains a syndicated health and fitness columnist for Knight Ridder Tribune. Her writing has also appeared in numerous health, fitness, and sports titles including *Health* magazine and *Alternative Medicine.* She enjoys rock climbing, snowboarding, trail running, hiking, backpacking, and basketball. She makes her home with her partner and two pups.